INTERMITTENT FASTING FOR WOMEN

The Secret To Effortlessly Lose Fat While Enjoying Life

TABLE OF CONTENTS

INTRODUCTION 3

INTERMITTENT FASTING FOR WOMEN: THE DO'S AND DON'TS 8

INTERMITTENT FASTING FOR FAT LOSS: GOOD OR BAD? 14

INTERMITTENT FASTING VS LOW CARB DIET? 18

FASTING FOR WEIGHT LOSS - LEARN HOW TO LOSE WEIGHT QUICKLY
BY DOING THIS! ……………………………………………………..………........21

INTERMITTENT FASTING METHODS: WHICH ONE IS RIGHT FOR YOU 25

BENEFITS OF INTERMITTENT FASTING 35

7 REASONS A FASTING DIET CAN MAKE YOU BURN MORE FAT 42

THINGS YOU PROBABLY DON'T KNOW ABOUT INTERMITTENT FASTING 45

INTERMITTENT FASTING FOR WOMEN. 47

5 DAY DIET PLAN - INTERMITTENT FASTING AND CHEATING FOR FASTER
WEIGHT LOSS ………………………………………………..……………....50

DO INTERMITTENT FASTING AND EXERCISING MESH? 52

INTERMITTENT FASTING RECIPE 57

INTRODUCTION

Intermittent fasting involves alternating periods of feast and famine in which you may eat as much as you like during the feasting but drink only water during the fast. The aim is to achieve the benefits of calorie reduction and for some, use it as vehicle to lose weight.

Intermittent fasting can be done over a number of days, in alternating 24 hour periods or daily. The first option requires you abstain from some or all meals on one or more days of the week. Daily fasting utilizes 24 hour periods of eating and fasting that begin an end at the same time each day, for example fast from Monday 6pm until Tuesday 6pm, eat as much as you like from Tuesday 6pm to Wednesday 6pm and repeat the process. During daily intermittent fasting there is a short period for eating, usually 4-6 hours within the 24 hour day during which you can eat as much as you like.

Some of the things that put people off are the fear that they will be extremely hungry and not stick to the plan or do not know how to fit it into their schedule. This is actually quite simple if you plan in advance you get eat your evening meal at pretty much the same time everyday but at an hour either side depending if on an intermittent fasting phase or an eating phase. Again with a little planning you can also accommodate socializing and eating out.

The main factor preventing many people from trying is the fear of being hungry. Although this does take a little will power and a slight degree of discomfort to begin with it is actually quite easy!

Intermittent fasting is a method that, if used properly, can greatly enhance your health and increase your weight loss. "Fasting" is a term used to describe a period of time when you go without eating, as is common in some religious practices. The term "intermittent" refers to the alternation of periods of eating and of fasting. So, intermittent fasting is basically a practice that involves eating within a certain time frame, and fasting in the time before and after. We all do this on a daily basis, since we are not eating when we are sleeping, but most of us do not "fast" for long enough periods of time to receive the benefits from it. Let me explain how you can alter your way of eating so that you can lose weight extremely easily without changing the types of food you eat or the amount of calories you eat.

To get the most out of intermittent fasting, you need to fast for at least 16 hours. At 16 hours and above, some of the amazing benefits of intermittent fasting kick in. An easy way to do this is to simply skip breakfast every morning. This is actually very healthy, but many people will try to tell you otherwise. By skipping breakfast, you are allowing your body to go into a caloric deficit, which will greatly increase the amount of fat you can burn and weight you can lose. Since your body is not busy digesting the food you ate, it has time to focus on burning your fat stores for energy and also for cleansing and detoxifying your body. If you find it difficult to skip breakfast, you can instead skip dinner, although I find this much more difficult. It really does not matter, but the goal is to extend the period of time you spend fasting and decrease the amount of time you spend eating. If you eat dinner at 6 o'clock at night, and don't eat until 10 the next morning, you have fasted for 16 hours. Longer is better, but you can see some pretty drastic changes from a daily 16 hour fast.

Losing weight is something that a lot of people all over the world are facing the problems of. But what most people fail to realise is that intermittent fasting is the best approach that you can use to really help you lose weight when you are struggling to get those pounds lost. Losing weight is and should not have to have hard. People make a big deal out of something that should be a slow and enjoyable process that everyone can enjoy.

Intermittent fasting and fasting in general is known throughout the world something that is very good for the health. But people in general do not want to go anywhere near it. People find that fasting is something that people will struggle with but the great thing about intermittent fasting is that you only do it on occasion. Plus a day doing fasting everyone in a while is a great way to get past that that plateau that you may have hit with losing the excess weight that you have on you.

The best way that you can apply intermittent fasting to your life is to start slowly, and gradually increase the time that you do it. This way you will allow your body to get used to the whole process and you will see the results without having to overwhelm yourself. So the key is to start slow and slowly increase the amount of time that you do it. Make sure that you do not do it more than once a week for maximum benefits.

Another thing that you need to take into consideration is that intermittent fasting is not the only thing that you are going to have to do to effectively lose weight. This has to be part of a big program that you are going to use in order to live a more healthy existence. You need to make sure that you diet is perfect, and you need to make sure that you are implementing a proper exercise routine into your life. Only when these things are perfect are you going to find that you will be seeing the long term results that you are after. Intermittent fasting is not an end to itself, but something that must be a part of a bigger strategy. This is the only way you are going to be successful.

Respective authors own all copyrights not held by the publisher.

The information herein is offered for informational purposes solely, and is universal as so. The presentation of the information is without contract or any type of guarantee assurance.

The trademarks that are used are without any consent, and the publication of the trademark is without permission or backing by the trademark owner. All trademarks and brands within this book are for clarifying purposes only and are owned by the owners themselves, not affiliated with this document.

INTERMITTENT FASTING FOR WOMEN: THE DO'S AND DON'TS

Over the last several years, there has been a lot of buzz around the concept of intermittent fasting (IF) and for good reason. Many people swear by intermittent fasting to decrease body fat, increase energy and focus, assist in detoxification, keep aging at bay, and even protect them against chronic disease. In fact, there is evidence to suggest that intermittent fasting can decrease the risk of certain diseases such as type 2 diabetes, cardiovascular disease, and even cancer.

In general, intermittent fasting is a way to manipulate the timing of your food intake to allow for periods of time spent in a fasting state which requires the body to turn to a different source of fuel – body fat. Not only that, but during times of fasting, blood glucose is lowered, growth hormone is triggered, hunger regulating hormones like leptin and ghrelin are normalized, detoxification becomes a focus, and the digestive system gets a rest and reset too. While our current society may find going large amounts of time without food to be against what we know, various cultures throughout history practice fasting regularly because of its amazing mind, body, and health benefits, not to mention our ancestors in the paleolithic area no doubt went through regular feasts and famines while hunting for food.

How does intermittent fasting work?

There are a few different methods of IF, all of which are effective, so it's more a matter of individual preference as to how someone incorporates it into their life.

Some examples include:

Scheduling one day per week to fast for 24 hours. The other 6 days have a normal food intake.

Schedule alternating days to eat very little (500-600 calories) and the other days have a normal food intake.

Scheduling a daily fast of 14-18 hours. This can be done by skipping breakfast or just condensing all 3 meals into an 6-10 hour window.

Do's and don'ts of intermittent fasting for women

Do keep tabs on your hormone health.

The biggest risk women have with intermittent fasting is with their hormones. Our hormones play a very delicate balancing act on a repeated 28-day cycle (on average). Sometimes the slightest change in our diet, health, mindset, environment, toxin exposure, or stress-level can cause hormonal imbalance to occur leading to further health issues down the road. If not done properly, intermittent fasting could easily become one of these triggers for hormonal imbalance because of the stress it can cause on your body.

It's not only the sex hormones that can be affected. Cortisol and thyroid hormones are also very important to monitor, especially if you have had past issues with thyroid disorders or adrenal fatigue.

Following the steps listed below will help tremendously in keeping your hormones balanced and stress level regulated. It is also very important to check on the state of your hormones before you even begin. If you are already dealing with a hormonal imbalance of any kind, addressing that issue will need to precede the intermittent fasting plan. The best way to do this is to test both your daily cortisol rhythm and your monthly hormonal cycle with a salivary collection.

Don't diet.

Ok, are you ready for the biggest reason why intermittent fasting DOESN'T work for women? Because we also try to diet at the same time! This is not the concept behind intermittent fasting and will ultimately either lead to bingeing, failure, or health and hormonal issues. During the period of time you are eating, you need to EAT. Eat a lot of really nutrient-dense, calorically-dense foods in that timeframe and do not try to be in a huge calorie deficit. This won't work. I like to think of intermittent fasting as a better, safer, smarter option to restricting calories. But, definitely never do both.

Do focus on fats.

In order to make sure you're not going into too big of a calorie deficit, your diet will need to consist primarily of healthy, nutrient-dense fats. These include fat from properly raised animals, unsweetened coconut and coconut oil, nuts and nut butters, pasture-raised butter or ghee, eggs, avocado and avocado oil, olives and olive oil, and grass-fed dairy products. When these foods become staples, you can rest assured that you will be getting enough nutrients and calories in your day prior to fasting.

Not only that, but switching to a high-fat diet will also ensure your fasting periods are stress-free, safe, and comfortable. With the reduction of carbohydrates and inclusion of a large amount of fat, your blood sugar will become extremely stable. Instead of being a rollercoaster (which is what happens to our blood sugar when we have excess carbohydrates in our diet), it will be more like small waves. When our bodies are on the rollercoaster route, there will be a dip in blood sugar a few hours after your last meal which brings on feelings of hunger. When no glucose is provided by way of a meal, cortisol – our stress hormone – will come to the rescue. So, now you're hungry, you're still fasting for another 5 hours, and your body senses a stressful event. Not good!

However, when you take a high-fat diet approach and become fat-adapted, that dip in blood sugar doesn't happen and the stressor isn't there because your body no longer relies on only glucose for energy. Your body has learned to run on fats – both dietary and stored body fat – instead of just waiting for the next meal. Now, not only are you not having feelings of hunger, but you're eliminating the stressful event! And, as we discussed above, the reason why intermittent fasting can be hard for women is because of the hormonal imbalance that can develop from the stress and cortisol response. Just by eating high-fat and plenty of food, we have eliminated that stressor!

Don't workout intensely.

At least for the first week or two until you know how intermittent will affect you. Once your body becomes adapted to this change, chances are workouts will actually feel better in the fasted state and you will begin to see improvements in your workouts. But, first you need to eliminate all added stressors while your body adapts and gets used to this new energy source (fat). Taking walks in nature or a really great yoga class will be the best way to get movement in during this transition time. After that, begin incorporating short HIIT sessions like jumping rope, sprinting, or heavy lifts in the gym and see how you feel. Remember, the end goal is to keep the stress level in the body at an all time low, thereby keeping your hormones in balance. Working out too intensely while your body is shifting energy sources will likely cause stress.

Don't make fat loss your main goal.

There are many success stories out there of people who have had complete body composition changes just by incorporating intermittent fasting. And it's true. It is a great tool for losing weight, getting leaner, and decreasing body fat. BUT, I don't think any female should do it just for that purpose. This is not the next way to obsess about your body and try to manipulate its size with food.

This is a therapeutic diet with amazing health benefits and should be viewed as such. Find a deeper purpose behind your dietary changes. Do you have brain fog or trouble concentrating? Intermittent fasting is great for brain health. Want to age well and live longer? Intermittent fasting has been shown to prolong lifespan and slow down the aging process. Need to get your blood lipids and cardiovascular markers in check? Intermittent fasting can bring those markers back in range without the use of medication.

Do start slow.

Intermittent fasting isn't something you need to dive into all or nothing for it to be effective. In fact, women may have better luck with easing their way into it. Spend 3-4 weeks becoming fat-adapted with a high fat diet first. Then, add in an intermittent fasting schedule a few days per week. For instance, try doing a 16/8 fast on Monday's and Thursday's and see how that feels. If you enjoy it, add in more days as you feel comfortable.

Don't continue if you feel bad.

This should go without saying, but obviously if you are feeling weak, tired, dizzy, or just don't like it, then don't do it! This is not something that will feel right for everyone, so pay attention, listen to your body, and always do what's right for you.

Do enlist the support of a professional.

As with any advice I give, I always recommend seeking the help of a professional to guide you through the changes you wish to make and support you along the way. This will make it easier to acknowledge what is right for YOU instead of just guessing. If you would like help in determining your individualized plan based on the state of your hormones, contact me for a free 15-minute case review.

INTERMITTENT FASTING FOR FAT LOSS: GOOD OR BAD?

As you may or may not have noticed, my title for this article includes a pretty sweet wordplay if I must say. Today I wanted to keep in mind the current time of year, Holidays. With that in mind, lets first take a q uick moment to be thankful for all or some of the following. Your car, your money, your ego, your image amongst friends and co workers, your shoes, your new cool tech gadget and all other cool things we consume. Or I guess we can say oh yea, lets take a chill pill on all that and be thankful for friends, family, loved ones, health, roofs over our head, great opportunities, great & abundant food, clean water, and an overall amazing community.

When we keep some of the above in mind it puts into perspective the stuff that we cover here on a weekly basis. Now I do not want to diminish the importance of this information at all, but more so put it in its proper place to make sure that we all realize it is not a matter of life and death but that it is something that can be utilized to increase your overall q uality of life in so many ways. And, as a result helping you bring more to the community you are a part of.

You may or may not have heard of Intermittent Fasting. It is a rather simple nutritional intervention that is being widely used and rather successfully might I add. It involves splitting your 24 hour day into two basic states or categories.

"Fast"-ed or "Fast"-ing state: (Anywhere from 18-48 hours)

"Fed" or "Feed"-ing state

Lets look at your fasting state first. The time ranges from 16 to 48 hours. I have played with the 16 hour state recently and have had a few experiences with the 24 hour fast as well.

To start this off you will typically have your dinner around lets say 7 or 8 pm. You would then enter your Fast for the next 16-18 hours for this example. So you would then wake up the next morning and potentially have your morning workout or get ready for work.

Side note: If you workout in the mornings I would not do this on workout days but 1 x per week. I prefer this on days of cardio only or 1 x per week of Resistance Training workouts.

You would then look at consuming your first meal around 11am - 1pm of that day.

Things to consider during your fast:

Potential Irritability

Increased need for water consumption

Greater ability to differentiate between false hunger and real hunger

Great caloric deficit and resetting of the body fat burning hormonal environment.

Need for consumption of Amino Acids during "fasting state" (specifically before and after morning "fasted state" workouts.)

Increased need for a delicious balanced meal when you come out of the fasted state.

Now lets look at the Feeding state.

This time period will only last the next 6-10 hours depending on your last meal for this day. During this time it is advisable to consume your main 3 meals. You still have breakfast aka (Break the Fast) just at a later time than your normal routine. It does not have to include your typical breakfast food but definitely can if that your thing.

Each meal will be of a decent size and will keep you going strong into the next day.

Things to consider during your Feed-ing or Fed state:

If you workout in the evening try keeping carbs moderate to low for pre-workout meals and then have a heavy carb meal after your evening workout to finish off the day and resulting fed state.

Don't go crazy on junk food for your first meal after the fast, that will totally erase all good coming from the fast.

Have the meals be of regular size and portions. Listen to your body and always allow for 15-20 minutes after eating to see if you need more food. That is how long it typically takes a meal to reach your tummy and its sensory receptors that signal hunger.

Pros and Cons of Intermittent Fasting + General Guidelines:

Pro: Create a massive caloric deficit

Pro: Increases fat & calorie burning

Pro: Increases ability to recognize true and false senses of hunger

Pro: You dont have to eat every 2-3 hours which can be a pain in the bum bum

Pro: Increased energy levels and metabolism

Cons: Women have a hard time with this diet

Cons: Takes a little getting used to

Cons: You may feel flat at times but that is not often reported

Guidelines:

I don't recommend this more than 2-4 x weekly with 2-3 days being the sweet spot for me at this point.

I recommend you try it out and see how you respond to it. Every body is different.

Have some amino acids on hand and be ready to take those during your morning hours and before/after workouts.

Lastly always consult with your medical doctor before attempting this.

There you have it guys. Go give this intermittent fasting for fat loss a try and share your thoughts and comments with me as it always helps me to make this stuff more simplified for you when I get those comments and q uestions.

INTERMITTENT FASTING VS LOW CARB DIET?

If you are looking for a way to reduce your body fat, going low carb is one of the popular diet choices. There a number of different versions of low carb diets , from the famous Atkins diet to The South Beach Diet. Low Carb Diets are not new, the concept was not invented by Dr Robert Atkins as many people seem to think. Low Carb diets even precede other US diet doctors such as Herman Tarnower and Herman Taller. Dieting Plans allowing you to eat meat, some dairy foods, salad and non-starchy vegetables,while restricting or banning foods containing sugar or starch were first promoted in the early 19th century by Jean Anthelme Brillat-Savarin. To this day the debate continues among Doctors and Nutritionists as to what is the best diet for us to follow and lose weight.

There is certainly evidence to show that initial weight loss while following a low carb diet does reduce body fat. In a recent study of popular diets (Gardner CD, Kiazand A, Alhassan S, et al. Comparison of the Atkins, Zone, Ornish, and LEARN diets for change in weight and related risk factors among overweight premenopausal women: the A TO Z Weight Loss Study: a randomized trial. JAMA 2007;297:969-77) The Atkins diet showed the best weight loss results over both a 2 month and a 6 month period. This is the information you seen mentioned in the media on a regular basis. However over a 12 month period the Atkins diet results were not so impressive, and was no more effective than the other diets in the study.

My own view based on my experience of trying low carb dieting is though effective in the short term, diets such as Atkins are not practical to follow in the long term. In my opinion, to lose body fat and control weight, the way we eat has to be possible to follow for the long term, not just for a few weeks. I have in the past done Atkins, The South Beach Diet, and Fat Flush. I have taken things from all of these diet plans, I use them as part of lifestyle today. I also have a greater understanding of the effect refined carbohydrates have on my body, but the simple fact remains I could not follow these plans as a long term lifestyle change.

This year I became a Retired Dieter. This means I no longer will refuse to eat the foods I enjoy. I have stopped listening to the media talk about the latest new diet and fat loss craze. All diets have a hook, but at the end of the day it comes down to one thing, one way or another we have to eat less. So what is the solution?

For me the effective way to lose body fat, and control my weight , is by using intermittent fasting. Intermittent Fasting is simply taking times of fast (no food) and working them into your lifestyle. You still eat every day, but you will incorporate a period of up to 24hrs without food into your day. Using Intermittent Fasting once or twice a week reduces body fat, yet still allows you to enjoy the foods you enjoy. On the days you are not fasting, you eat normally. Following the I.F. lifestyle I am still cutting carbs from my diet. I am actually cutting carbs for the equivalent of 2 full days per week.

We could debate the theory, but I like to work on results. In my first 7 weeks of using Intermittent Fasting for weight loss, I have reduced my body fat by 12% and lost 24lbs. In my 14 years of trying different diet plans, I have never had results that compare to these. The other main point is, unlike my experience of low carb diets, I have not felt restricted with Intermittent Fasting,I have not had any cravings for specific foods like I did with Low Carb dieting because no foods are off limits. Why do I feel that intermittent fasting is something I can use as long term after only 7 weeks? The answer is because on any diet I have tried in the past, I would always have days where I felt i was restricted, so the diet became difficult, and that is on the diets that I managed to stick to for 7 weeks! The difference with Intermittent Fasting is, it isn't a diet, because no foods are off limits. Once you have completed once fast, you know from that day forward, you can incorporate it into your lifestyle, how you do that, and how often you do it, is up to you, that is the great thing about Intermittent Fasting, it adapts to your lifestyle, in the past when you went on a diet, how often did it dominate your life? This again is a prime example why diets fail.

So my suggestion is if you are looking to reduce your body fat, and think you should reduce your carbs, try Intermittent Fasting. Become a Retired Dieter, and let me know how you get on.

FASTING FOR WEIGHT LOSS - LEARN HOW TO LOSE WEIGHT

QUICKLY BY DOING THIS!

Fasting has been used by many religions for penitence, to show their faith, or a chance for spiritual contemplation. It has also been used historically in politics to convey their views or as a kind of protest. Fasting involves abstaining from food or drink for a specified period of time. Nowadays a lot of people used fasting to cleanse the body of harmful toxins, as a way to lose weight, and for other medical reasons.

Fasting has become a popular weight loss program and differs with each diet. Certain fasting diets only allow liq uids like water, juice, or tea, or eating raw foods for a certain length of time; others restrict food on alternating days; and there are some that significantly reduce calorie intake without doing away with food. However, due to certain health risks, fasting for weight loss should be done by following several steps to make sure that it will be effective and healthy for your body. Below are some of the basics steps to safely lose weight while fasting:

Use intermittent fasting which involves fasting for a certain length of time (like fasting for 20 hours in a day and then eating food for the remaining 4 hours), or eating normally in alternate days.

Pay careful attention to the calories you will be consuming during off times when fasting. Make sure that every calorie counts by eating lean proteins, complex carbohydrates, and healthy fats in order to give your body the energy it needs to support you during fasting periods.

Limit your exercises to light physical activities during fasting. Intense workouts might only cause you injury, making it harder for you t maintain your fast.

Tune in to your body and look for another weight loss program suitable for you than going on a fast.

Fasting might not work for you if you are having a headache, get sick, fatigued, or have trouble concentrating.

Set a definite time period for fasting to make it easier for you to maintain it while on a diet.

Consult your doctor first to make sure there are no medical issues that will prevent you from fasting.

Another effective way to get the most of fasting for weight loss is by including some light exercises regularly to at least 30 minutes. Light exercises may be walking, swimming, biking, and even stretching. These activities should be easy and enjoyable for you to do. It is not recommended that you engage in strenuous exercises while fasting.

Various Reasons Why People Fast:

For detoxifying the body - the body goes into ketosis when you abstain from eating for a day or two. Ketosis happens when the body burns fat instead because there is not enough carbohydrates to burn for energy. This helps in detoxification since most of the toxins in the body are stored in fats.

For fast weight loss

For religious or spiritual reasons

For medical reasons - fasting is necessary before surgery and for accurate readings of medical laboratory tests like blood sugar and cholesterol levels.

For treating disease - fasting is an effective way to treat medical issues like depression, arthritis, heart disease, lupus, ulcerative colitis, Crohn's disease, psoriasis, eczema, and lowers blood pressure.

For longer life - fasting and calorie-restricted diet helps to extend the lifespan of individuals by delaying the onset of age-related diseases. Healthy eating habits and periodic fasting can help people live longer.

For psychological reasons - fasting is also often used to help people deal with stress and depression.

Two Major Types of Fasting:

There are 2 methods of fasting and each one complement the other and can be combined to achieve the ideal weight you desire in addition to improving your health.

1. Water or Juice Fasting - This method involves consuming only water or liq uid juices, most preferably those made from fresh fruits and vegetables. This type of fasting is also safer because it gives the body the nutrients it needs for proper functioning.

2. Intermittent Fasting - This second method of fasting involves eating and fasting on alternate days.

How Fasting Works:

During fasting, the metabolic rate slows down to preserve energy and the body will make the adjustments by reducing your appetite. On the first day of fasting, the body will make use of glycogen (small q uantities of glucose stored in the liver and muscles) to keep it functioning properly. When the body runs out of carbohydrates to convert to energy, it burns fat instead. After fasting for several days, protein is broken down and converted to glucose.

How Safe Is Fasting for Weight Loss?

A day or two of fasting is generally safe for healthy people as long as they maintain sufficient intake of liq uids.

Fasting is not safe for pregnant or breastfeeding women and for people who have health issues like malnutrition, liver or kidney problems, diabetics, cardiac arrhythmia, and those with compromised immune functioning.

Individuals who are on medications are also advised to refrain from fasting.

Advantages of Fasting:

Helps control hunger and

Provides anti-aging effect

Improves concentration and might even help in building new brain cells

Promotes healthy change in diet and lifestyle

INTERMITTENT FASTING METHODS: WHICH ONE IS RIGHT FOR YOU

We've all heard of the latest fad diets: The no-fat, all-fat, cabbage-soup, six-small-meals, raw-veggies-no-dressing, gluten-free eating plans supposedly proven to help you lose weight fast.

What if we told you that the answer to losing weight, improving body composition, and feeling better isn't about dieting, but instead skipping meals every once in a while? For some, intermittent fasting, or going a longer period of time — usually between 14 and 36 hours — with few to no calories, can be a lot easier than you may think. And the benefits might be worth it. If you think about it, all of us "fast" every single day — we just call it sleeping. Intermittent fasting just means extending that fasting period, and being a bit more conscious of your eating schedule overall. But is it right for you? And which method is best?

The Science of Fasting

As far back as the 1930s, scientists have been exploring the benefits of reducing calories by skipping meals. During that time, one American scientist found that significantly reducing calories helped mice live longer, healthier lives. More recently, researches have found the same in fruit flies, roundworms and monkeys. Studies have also shown that decreasing calorie consumption by 30 to 40 percent (regardless of how it's done) can extend life span by a third or more. Plus, there's data to suggest that limiting food intake may reduce the risk of many common diseases. Some believe fasting may also increase the body's responsiveness to insulin, which regulates blood sugar and helps control hunger.

The five most common methods of intermittent fasting try to take advantage of each of these benefits. But different methods will yield better results for different people. "If you're going to force yourself to follow a certain method, it's not going to work," says trainer and fitness expert Nia Shanks. "Choose a method that makes your life easier," she says. Otherwise, it's not sustainable and the benefits of your fasting may be short-lived.

So what's the first step in getting started? Each method has its own guidelines for how long to fast and what to eat during the "feeding" phase. Below, you'll find the five most popular methods and the basics of how they work. Keep in mind, intermittent fasting isn't for everyone. Those with health conditions of any kind should check with their doctor before changing up their usual routine. Note that personal goals and lifestyle are key factors to consider when choosing a fasting method.

Intermittent Fasting: 5 Methods

1. Leangains

How It Works: Fast for 14 (women) to 16 (men) hours each day, and then "feed" for the remaining eight to 10 hours. During the fasting period, you consume no calories. However, black coffee, calorie-free sweeteners, diet soda and sugar-free gum are permitted. (A splash of milk in your coffee won't hurt, either.) Most practitioners will find it easiest to fast through the night and into the morning. They usually break the fast roughly six hours after waking up. This schedule is adaptable to any person's lifestyle, but maintaining a consistent feeding window time is important.

Otherwise, hormones in the body can get thrown out of whack and make sticking to the program harder, Berkhan says.

What and when you eat during the feeding window also depends on when you work out. On days you exercise, carbs are more important than fat. On rest days, fat intake should be higher. Protein consumption should be fairly high every day, though it will vary based on goals, gender, age, body fat and activity levels. Regardless of your specific program, whole, unprocessed foods should make up the majority of your calorie intake. However, when there isn't time for a meal, a protein shake or meal replacement bar is acceptable (in moderation).

Pros: For many, the highlight of this program is that on most days, meal frequency is irrelevant. You can really eat whenever you want to within the eight-hour "feeding" period. That said, most people find breaking it up into three meals easier to stick to (since we're typically already programmed to eat this way).

Cons: Even though there is flexibility in when you eat, Leangains has pretty specific guidelines for what to eat, especially in relation to when you're working out. The strict nutrition plan and scheduling meals perfectly around workouts can make the program a bit tougher to adhere to. (You can learn more about the specifics — as well as when to time these meals — directly from Leangains here and here.)

2. Eat Stop Eat

Started by: Brad Pilon

Best for: Healthy eaters looking for an extra boost.

It's all about moderation: You can still eat whatever you want, but maybe not as much of it. A slice of birthday cake is OK, but the whole cake isn't.

How It Works: Fast for 24 hours once or twice per week. During the 24 hour fast, which creator Brad Pilon prefers to call a "24 break from eating," no food is consumed, but you can drink calorie-free beverages. After the fast is over, you then go back to eating normally. "Act like you didn't fast," Pilon says. "Some people need to finish the fast at a normal mealtime with a big meal, while others are OK ending the fast with an afternoon snack. Time it however works best for you, and adjust your timing as your schedule changes," he says.

The main rationale? Eating this way will reduce overall calorie intake without really limiting what you're able to eat — just how often, according to Eat Stop Eat. It's important to note that incorporating regular workouts, particularly resistance training, is key to succeeding on this plan if weight loss or improved body composition are goals.

Pros: While 24 hours may seem like a long time to go without food, the good news is that this program is flexible. You don't have to go all-or-nothing at the beginning. Go as long as you can without food the first day and gradually increase fasting phase over time to help your body adjust.

Pilon suggests starting the fast when you are busy, and on a day where you have no eating obligations (like a work lunch or happy hour).

Another perk? There are no "forbidden foods," and no counting calories, weighing food or restricting your diet, which makes it a bit easier to follow. That said, this isn't a free-for-all. "You still have to eat like a grown-up," Pilon says. It's all about moderation: You can still eat whatever you want, but maybe not as much of it. (A slice of birthday cake is OK, he says, but the whole cake isn't.)

Cons: Going 24 hours without any calories may be too difficult for some — especially at first. Many people struggle with going extended periods of time with no food, citing annoying symptoms including headaches, fatigue, or feeling cranky or anxious (though these side effects can dimish over time). The long fasting period can also make it more tempting to binge after a fast. This can be easily fixed… but it takes a lot of self-control, which some people lack.

3. The Warrior Diet

Started by: Ori Hofmekler

Best for: People who like following rules. The devoted.

How It Works: Warriors-in-training can expect to fast for about 20 hours every day and eat one large meal every night. What you eat and when you eat it within that large meal is also key to this method. The philosophy here is based on feeding the body the nutrients it needs in sync with circadian rhythms and that our species are "nocturnal eaters, inherently programmed for night eating."

The fasting phase of The Warrior Diet is really more about "undereating." During the 20-hour fast, you can eat a few servings of raw fruit or veggies, fresh juice, and a few servings of protein, if desired. This is supposed to maximize the Sympathetic Nervous System's "fight or flight" response, which is intended to promote alertness, boost energy, and stimulate fat burning.

The four-hour eating window — which Hofmekler refers to as the "overeating" phase — is at night in order to maximize the Parasympathetic Nervous System's ability to help the body recuperate, promoting calm, relaxation and digestion, while also allowing the body to use the nutrients consumed for repair and growth. Eating at night may also help the body produce hormones and burn fat during the day, according to Hofmekler. During these four hours, the order in which you eat specific food groups matters, too. Hofmelker says to start with veggies, protein and fat. After finishing those groups, only if you are still hungry should you tack on some carbohydrates.

Pros: Many have gravitated toward this diet because the "fasting" period still allows you to eat a few small snacks, which can make it easier to get through. As the methodology explains (and the "success stories" section of The Warrior Diet website supports), many practitioners also report increased energy levels and fat loss.

Cons: Even though it's nice to eat a few snacks rather than go without any food for 20-plus hours, the guidelines for what you need to eat (and when) can be hard to follow long-term. The strict schedule and meal plan may also interfere with social gatherings. Additionally, eating one main meal at night — while following strict guidelines of what to eat, and in what order — can be tough. It's especially hard for those who prefer not to eat large meals late in the day.

4. Fat Loss Forever

How It Works: Not completely satisfied with the IF diets listed above? This method takes the best parts of Eat Stop Eat, The Warrior Diet and Leangains, and combines it all into one plan. You also get one cheat day each week (yay!) — followed by a 36-hour fast (which may be not-so-yay for some). After that, the remainder of the seven-day cycle is split up between the different fasting protocols.

Romaniello and Go suggest saving the longest fasts for your busiest days, allowing you to focus on being productive. The plan also includes training programs (using bodyweight and free weights) to help participants reach maximum fat loss in the simplest way possible.

Pros: According to the founders, while everyone is technically fasting every day — during the hours when we're not eating — most of us do so haphazardly, which makes it harder to reap the rewards. Fat Loss Forever offers a seven-day schedule for fasting so that the body can get used to this structured timetable and reap the most benefit from the fasting periods. (Plus, you get a full cheat day. And who doesn't love that?)

Cons: On the flip side, if you have a hard time handling cheat days the healthy way, this method might not be for you. Additionally, because the plan is pretty specific and the fasting/feeding schedule varies from day to day, this method can be a bit confusing to follow. (However, the plan does come with a calendar, noting how to fast and exercise each day, which may make it easier.)

5. UpDayDownDay Diet (aka The Alternate-Day Diet or Alternate-Day Fasting)

How It Works: This one's easy: Eat very little one day, and eat like normal the next. On the low-calorie days, that means one fifth of your normal calorie intake. Using 2,000 or 2,500 calories (for women and men, respectively) as a guide, "fasting" (or "down") day should be 400 to 500 calories. Followers can use this tool to figure out how many calories to consume on "low-calorie" days.

To make "down" days easier to stick to, Johnson recommends opting for meal replacement shakes. They're fortified with essential nutrients and you can sip them throughout the day rather than split into small meals. However, meal replacement shakes should only be used during the first two weeks of the diet — after that, you should start eating real food on "down" days. The next day, eat like normal. Rinse and repeat! (Note: If working out is part of your routine, you may find it harder to hit the gym on the lower calorie days. It may be smart to keep any workouts on these days on the tamer side, or save sweat sessions for your normal calorie days.)

Pros: This method is all about weight loss, so if that's your main goal, this is one to take a closer look at. On average, those who cut calories by 20 to 35 percent see a loss of about two and a half pounds per week, according to the Johnson UpDayDownDay Diet website.

Cons: While the method is pretty easy to follow, it can be easy to binge on the "normal" day. The best way to stay on track is planning your meals ahead of time as often as possible. Then you're not caught at the drive-through or all-you-can-eat buffet with a grumbling belly.

It takes our bodies time to adjust, and some req uire more than others. "Be cautious at first, and start slowly [with a shorter fast]," Shanks recommends.

While these five methods are the most well-known in terms of integrating periods of fasting into your eating schedule, there are many other similar philosophies based on meal timing. For those who prefer a more fluid, less rigid method, there's also the concept of eating intuitively. Primal Diet proponent Mark Sisson is a supporter of the Eat WHEN (When Hunger Ensues Naturally) method, where dieters simply eat whenever their bodies ask them to. However, some believe this can also lead to overeating or overconsumption of calories, since our bodies' hunger-induced choices may be more caloric than otherwise.

Of course, fasting — regardless of the method — isn't for everyone. If you have any medical conditions or special dietary req uirements, it's smart to consult a doctor before giving intermittent fasting a shot. Anyone who tries it should also plan to be highly self-aware while fasting. If it's not agreeing with you, or if you need to eat a little something to hold you over, that's just fine. It takes our bodies time to adjust, and some require more than others. Keep in mind that hormones can make it harder for women to follow a fasting plan than for men. "Be cautious at first, and start slowly [with a shorter fast]," Shanks recommends. If it doesn't make you feel better, try something different, or accept the fact that maybe fasting isn't for you.

If you do give fasting a try, keep these general tips in mind:

Drink plenty of water. Staying well hydrated will make the fasting periods much easier to get through, Pilon says.

Fast overnight. Throw yourself a bone and aim to fast through the night. That way, you're (hopefully) sleeping during at least eight of those hours.

Rewire your thought process. "Think of fasting as taking a break from eating," Pilon says, not as a period of deprivation. It can be a way to break up the monotony of worrying about what you need to eat next and when. This is the mindset that will allow you do follow a fasting plan long-term, he says.

Overcommit. It may seem counterintuitive, but the best plan is often to start when you're busy — not on a day when you'll be sitting on the couch wanting to snack.

BENEFITS OF INTERMITTENT FASTING

Intermittent fasting has become quite the phenomenon these days. Recent studies showed that people who tried it have lost weight, increased health, and believed to have a long lifespan. Basically, intermittent fasting is a pattern of eating that alternates between periods of fasting, usually consuming only water, and non-fasting, usually eating anything a person want no matter how fattening. In other words, a person can eat anything he wants during a 24-hour period and fast for the next 24 hours. This approach to weight control seems to be supported by science, as well as religious and cultural practices around the globe. Adherents of intermittent fasting claim that this practice is a way to become more circumspect about food.

There are many different popular intermittent fasts and hundreds more possible variations. There are two kinds of intermittent fasts that are most basic and freq uently used. First is the daily fasting in which the person only gets to eat once every 20-28 hours within a 4-hour period. The second is fasting for 1-3x a week, also called alternate day fasting, in which a person eats anything he wants on one day and fast the whole of next day.

Intermittent fasting has many beneficial effects as tested on animals like rodents and primates. One study found that there has been a "reduced serum glucose and insulin levels and increased resistance of neurons in the brain to excitotoxic stress". In 2008, a study on intermittent fasting showed that lifespan increases of 40.4% and 56.6% in C. elegans for alternate day (24 hour) and two-of-each-three day (48 hour) fasting, respectively, as compared to an ad libitum diet. And a 2009 study showed that intermittent fasting on rats improved long-term survival after chronic heart failure via pro-angiogenic, anti-apoptotic and anti-remodeling effects.

Researchers caution that only a few studies have been done on humans who are practicing intermittent fasts. The effects of exercise and meal freq uency on body composition are an interesting but largely unexplored area of research. However, there are some positive results. Just last month, the Proceedings of the National Academy of Sciences published a study showing that reducing calories 30% a day increased the memory function of the elderly. In 2007, the journal Free Radical Biology & Medicine published a study that showed asthma patients who fasted had fewer symptoms, better airway function and a decrease in the markers of inflammation in the blood than those who didn't fast.

Everyone always wonders what the next big secret in the dieting industry is... Specifically, people want to burn fat and build muscle while putting in as little effort as possible. They want it all, and sometimes that's asking a little too much. At-least with most programs.

But what If I told you there were programs ahead of the entire industry that could do that? Enter intermittent fasting.

Let's kill a highly perpetuated myth before we move on to the benefits of intermittent fasting.

Breakfast is the most important meal of the day:

That myth is easily killed. Those who engage in regular fasting (often goes from sleep to lunch, meaning skipping breakfast) report increased focus, increased energy levels and better mood while fasting. Looking for your new coffee? You've found one that burns fat and gives you energy.

Eating 6 meals a day speeds up the metabolism:

If you are consuming the same number of calories and have the same macronutrient distribution (primarily talking about protein), consuming those calories and nutrients between 6 meals and 1 makes near 0 difference. Because at the end of the day with either method, if I cut calories, there will be the same caloric deficit, and if I add calories, there will be the same surplus!

And if there was a difference, I am inclined to believe that it is in favor of the fasting method.

By increasing insulin sensitivity, intermittent fasting can make sure when you are eating the calories are getting driven directly into your muscles! And when you aren't fasting the increased adrenaline/noradrenaline will give you energy and burn fat!

In the most simple sense, intermittent fasting is rotating between periods of eating, and periods of not eating. I'll list the benefits below, but the general reasoning behind participating in Intermittent fasting(IF) is that many people respond very well to eating most of their calories in less meals, especially while dieting.

This allows for hunger control, insulin sensitivity (read: muscle building) and more time for burning fat (increased adrenaline/noradrenaline).

Methods:

You might fast through your sleep and into the afternoon, and then have a window of eating that lasts a few hours. In this period you would also have the workout.

Or it could mean that you wake up and eat a large meal, and fast late into the day until second/last meal.

Be smart and efficient, choose a program that gets you results with researched efficient methods. Either way the responsibility is taken at your leisure, but to squeeze the most results out of any method you choose, do your research and listen to your body.

Possible Benefits of Intermittent fasting:

*Increased Insulin sensitivity/nutrient portioning, makes for a great way to build muscle without gaining fat!

*Increased adrenaline/noradrenaline, meaning more time spent burning fat!

*Reduced appetite and hunger, possibility of feeling full due to eating all calories in fewer meals

Example:

If you're allotted 1800 calories on your diet, would you rather eat 2 900 calorie meals, or 6 300 calorie meals?

*Increased energy and focus

And so much more...

This is everything you want in a diet. We want to reap all the benefits while building the body of our dreams and this is the perfect way to do it! This is how you accomplish the number one goal of the fitness industry... burning fat while building muscle!

A little disclosure:

Intermittent fasting is way ahead of the rest of the industry. It goes against a lot of the mainstream myths that are currently being perpetuated and that you might believe. But then again, we have to ask ourselves, do we want mainstream results? Or do we want to be above average, uniq ue and at the top? I know my answer.

Other Benefits Of Intermittent Fasting

Muscle Building Vegetables

Numerous studies have shown that there truly are a number of awesome benefits that come with incorporating intermittent fasting into your daily or weekly dietary routine. One the most important benefits of intermittent fasting has to do with improving overall wellness and triggering anti-aging effects in the body. Intermittent fasting has been shown to trigger a process called autophagy. This is where cells begin their clean up and removal of harmful waste materials such as free radicals. This is also the time when cells will repair themselves, making themselves stronger. Autophagy has been shown to help fight the aging process as well as help maintain lean muscle tissue.

An Improvement of Insulin Sensitivity

One study collected two groups of subjects and placed one on an intermittent fasting diet and another on a traditional diet. The study showed that those volunteers who were on the intermittent fasting diet had a significant improvement in insulin sensitivity and glucose uptake. Insulin sensitivity is extremely important post-workout as this is when your body will be looking for the necessary nutrients to build muscle.

Reduction of Bodyfat

Another study found that human and animal subjects that were placed on an alternate-day fasting program experienced decreased body fat, improved insulin sensitivity, decreased blood pressure, and increased glucose uptake.

For bodybuilders and those looking to increase lean muscle tissue, this next study is very important. A team at the University of Virginia concluded that intermittent fasting triggered an increase in levels of human growth hormone in the body. ("Augmented growth hormone (GH) secretory burst freq uency and amplitude mediate enhanced GH secretion during a two-day fast in normal men." 1992. Para. 1)

Overall Benefits of Intermittent Fasting

To sum it up, a variety of studies have shown that Intermittent Fasting, when followed as recommended, is capable of providing the following benefits:

Improved immune system

Fighting the aging process

Securing lean muscle tissue

Reducing body fat

Increased levels of HGH

Decreased blood pressure

7 REASONS A FASTING DIET CAN MAKE YOU BURN MORE FAT

Just to clarify when we talk about fasting diet what I actually mean is intermittent fasting where you only fast for 24 hour 2 or 3 times a week. This method is becoming a very popular way to help burn body fat in a short period time and to help maintain your weight loss for life.

That said here are 7 ways this type of fasting can help you burn body fat quickly

1. Your Fat Burning Hormones are increased

HGH (Human Growth Hormone) is the most important fat hormone in our body. When we are a fasted state the production of this hormone is increased resulting in higher amounts of fat being burned. Fasting also allows the insulin levels in our body to reduce so you burn fat and not store it

2. You have lots more fat burning enzymes

When you are producing more fat burning hormones then you need more fat burning enzymes to help them do their job properly. The two most important enzymes that assist in this process are Adipose tissue HSL and Muscle Tissue LPL. Simply explained the HSL enzyme encourages your fat cells to release fat for energy to be used in your muscles and the LPL enzyme has the job of getting your muscles to soak up the fat so it can be burnt for fuel. Fasting increases the release of both these enzymes therefore creating a fantastic fat burning environment.

3. You actually will burn more calories when fasting

I have to admit I was not sure about this claim at first but after a few weeks of my fasting diet I found myself having extra energy and being more alert and awake on my fast days. The reason for this is that short term fasting (12-72hrs) actually boosts your metabolism and adrenaline levels. This combination results in extra calories being used and as we all know the more calories you burn the faster you can lose weight.

4. Instead of burning sugar you now burn more fat

When you have a meal your body will first burn the carbs then the fat from your food. If you can't burn off this fat in few hours after this food then its going to be stored as fat. When you are fasting there is no other energy source in your body so it has to burn body fat and not the sugar in your blood put there by the food.

5. You can understand what triggers you to eat.

When I made a decision to fast what surprised me most was how aware I became of the triggers and habits that made me eat badly. A lot of my unhealthy eating was down to routine and certain situations and by being able to see these more clearly I started to break these bad habits. Knowing why and what causes you to eat certain foods is an important step to stopping this reaction can help build better habits.

6. Get control back over what you eat.

By doing short fasts you do feel better about yourself and get a feeling of accomplishment. If you have issues with food then this positive response can help you build a positive relationship with food again. Being in control of what you eat will make sure you are not as vulnerable to eating all the bad foods that cause to put on weight.

7. You can still enjoy all the foods you like.

Short term fasting allows you to burn fat and ultimately lose weight while still enjoying foods you like. The discipline of fasting means on the other days you can have the foods you enjoy but without the guilt and still lose weight.

With this type of freedom in your diet you are far more likely to stick to the plan because you don't feel restricted. Most people fail to hit their goals because they stop too soon so being able to be consistent over time is the difference between failure and success.

THINGS YOU PROBABLY DON'T KNOW ABOUT INTERMITTENT FASTING

About a month ago, I received an email from world-renown nutrition and fat loss expert, John Berardi. The headline of the email, "New Book: Experiments with Intermittent Fasting" immediately piq ued my interest. Intrigued by the idea of a new and interesting online weight loss program, I decided to pursue this idea a little more.

As an ever-hungry student of exercise and nutrition, I have studied and tried many different approaches to eating and training over the years, from fat loss to muscle building to increased athletic performance, and everywhere in between. Though I had heard about intermittent fasting and its claimed benefits (though somewhat radical in reputation), I had never really looked into it much.

However, always interested in what Dr. Berardi has to say, I decided to check out his new e-book. About three hours later, I finally stood up from my chair after devouring the entire book in one sitting! Here are just a few things that I learned about intermittent fasting:

1. Intermittent Fasting (also referred to as I.F.), though given a pretty cool and somewhat exotic name, is simply the term that nutrition experts give to going certain extended periods of time without eating.

2. We all practice a form of intermittent fasting practically every day...when we sleep! That's right. From your last meal of the evening until

your first meal the next day, you are practicing a form of intermittent fasting.

3. Though there is still lots of research left to do on intermittent fasting, some potential benefits include reduced blood pressure, reduced risk of some cancers, increased metabolic rate (think increased fat burning potential), and improved blood sugar control and cardiovascular functioning.

4. There are many different styles of I.F. programs. Some include one or more full fasting days (that's at least 24 hours straight without food) while some follow a less dramatic approach, such as the Leangains approach (16-hour fast/8-hour feed).

5. Intermittent fasting is not for the faint of heart. Before considering I.F., you should first understand the basic fundamentals for healthy weight loss and good nutrition. That being said, if you are a more advanced dieter and exerciser looking for a new and challenging way to burn fat, I.F. might be worth checking out. Just be aware that it will take sound planning and discipline to follow some of these approaches.

So there's a brief overview of intermittent fasting, as well as just a few of the topics that are contained in Dr. Berardi's new book, "Experiments with Intermittent Fasting." I hope I have provided enough information to rouse your interest in this intriguing, yet somewhat unusual, approach to health and fat loss.

INTERMITTENT FASTING FOR WOMEN.

By now, you may have heard of some of the incredible benefits of intermittent fasting. Things like a higher metabolism, weight loss, and increased energy, among many other benefits, can all be experienced, and I'll explore them further below. As soon as I heard about this amazing practice, I thought it would be something that I could simply incorporate into my lifestyle to aid my health and I began doing it right away. It wasn't long after that I found some information explaining how women must be careful with this practice because it can actually cause hormonal imbalance and even lead to fertility issues. So if you are a woman and intermittent fasting interests you, here's what you need to know.

advertisement - learn more

What Is Intermittent Fasting?

First off, you may have no idea what intermittent fasting even is, so let me explain. The process of intermittent fasting involves restricting the eating period to an 8-10 hour window, so that you are going between 12 and 16 hours or more with absolutely no food in your system. Water, herbal tea, and black coffee are fine, however.

While this may sound really difficult to achieve, especially if you are someone who likes to eat at night, consider this: If you normally have dinner at 7pm and don't eat anything until 10am the next day, you are already doing it, because you are going 15 hours without food. Basically cutting out that late night snack might be all you need to make intermittent fasting a part of your routine.

Medical studies have shown that intermittent fasting can:

Increase energy

Improve cognitive function, memory, and focus

Make us less insulin resistant

Increases the immune system, improves heart health, lowers diabetes risk

Increases the production of brain neurotropic growth factor, a protein that promotes neuron growth, helping to make us more resistant to neurological stress and thus making us less susceptible to neurodegenerative diseases.

So, as you can see, this simple daily practice can absolutely be a great addition to your lifestyle.

Women and Intermittent Fasting

As mentioned above, intermittent fasting can have adverse effects on women and their hormones if not done correctly. Intermittent fasting is relatively new to the mainstream medical system and unfortunately, to date there haven't been any conclusive studies conducted on the effects of intermittent fasting on women specifically. There have been several animal studies, however, and research has shown that after two weeks of intermittent fasting, female rats stopped having menstrual cycles and their ovaries shrunk. They also experienced more insomnia than the males who were also part of the study.

Women are much more sensitive to starvation signals than men, and if the body senses it is being starved, it will ramp up the production of the hunger hormones, leptin and ghrelin. When women experience that feeling of insatiable hunger after not eating enough, what they are actually feeling are these hormones. This is how a woman's body protects the potential fetus, even if a woman is not pregnant. Sometimes, we ignore these signals, but this can cause us to binge eat later, and the process of starving and then bingeing is in itself a vicious cycle that can throw your hormones out of balance and thus halt the ovulation process.

A safe solution for women who want the benefits of intermittent fasting without the potential risks is to start off with something called Crescendo fasting.

The basic rules of crescendo fasting are as follows:

Fast on 2-3 nonconsecutive days per week (e.g. Monday, Wednesday and Saturday).

On the days of your fast, choose yoga, stretching, or light cardio for exercise.

Eat normally on days you are practicing strength training or high intensity interval workout days.

Fast for 12-16 hours on your fasting days

Stay hydrated.

After two weeks, add on another day of fasting if you wish.

You may want to consider taking 5-8 grams of branched chain amino acid supplements (BCAAs), which have few calories but provide fuel to the muscles. and can help take the edge off any hunger and fatigue you may experience.

If you have tried and failed at intermittent fasting before, maybe the crescendo fasting style is better for you! Every body is different and has different needs, so experiment to discover what works best for you.

5 DAY DIET PLAN - INTERMITTENT FASTING AND CHEATING FOR FASTER WEIGHT LOSS

The accepted method for faster weight loss has changed. Gone are the days of reducing your calorie intake and keeping it low. This out-of-date method leads to misery and a slow metabolism. Research today is focused on constantly shifting your calorie intake to keep your body confused so it never adapts to your diet. This method keeps your metabolism high and gives you the best and fastest weight loss possible. This article shares a 5 day diet plan that shows you how to use intermittent fasting and cheating days to burn off the fat in record time.

Faster Weight Loss

By constantly altering your diet you stay one step ahead of your body and it never has time to adapt to your diet. To do this follow the recommendations below.

Day 1: Start with a Cheat Day. A high calorie day creates the right hormonal conditions inside your body to support rapid weight loss. The key to understanding why this works is to understand that weight loss is highly dependent on hormones. One in particular, leptin, is nicknamed the "anti-starvation" hormone and it is the one most responsible for slowing your metabolism when you fast or severely reduce your calorie intake for more than a few days. When you cheat or overeat you boost your leptin levels and this in turn keeps your metabolism high.

Day 2: Fast or near fast day. On this day keep your calories very low. The conditions are right inside your body for rapid weight loss thanks to Day

1 so use this day to drastically create a calorie deficit. You can further this deficit with exercise on this day.

Day 3: Low calorie day. Though not as severe as Day 2, this day you will keep your calories at a low level. This will vary for different people but generally the low 1,000 calories per day range for women and the mid 1,000 calorie per day range for men.

Day 4: Moderate carbohydrate day: You want to give your body a small energy boost on this day, which can also add back some of the lost glycogen storage (basically carbohydrate storage) into your muscles. Eat a diet with approximately 40% carbohydrates, 30% protein, and 30% fats.

Day 5: Protein only day: This day you will completely deplete your carbohydrate storage again to keep your body confused and also prepare for your next Cheat Day the following day. On this day exercise to further deplete carbohydrate storage.

Repeat this cycle up to 5 times then take a break. Check with your doctor before beginning the diet to be sure it is safe for you and then enjoy the results.

DO INTERMITTENT FASTING AND EXERCISING MESH?

"While you may shed more fat when exercising on an IF diet, you may lose more muscle, too."

Before you get too excited, consider this: "When glycogen is in short supply, your body also reverts to breaking down protein — your muscles' building blocks — for fuel," Pritchett says. So, while you may shed more fat when exercising on an intermittent fasting (or IF) diet, you may lose more muscle, too. If you're heading out on a long run, but haven't eaten any carbs, your body might start burning protein within a couple of hours.

That won't just thwart how much weight you can bench press or how toned your butt looks — it will also slow your metabolism, which can make losing weight more difficult in the long run. In an effort to prevent starvation, your body adapts to the number calories you give it. So if you're freq uently making drastic cuts to your calorie intake, your body will eventually adjust — burning fewer calories per day to ensure you have enough energy left to stay upright, breathing and healthy, Pritchett says.

In one small study from the Pennington Biomedical Research Center, after a group of men and women fasted every other day for 22 days, their resting metabolic rates (how many calories they burned each day by simply living), had dropped by five percent, or 83 calories. Not exactly ideal for any exercise plan that's supposed to end in weight loss.

Plus, if you've ever tried to power through a tough workout with a growling stomach, you know that working out on empty is just plain hard. If your glycogen or blood sugar levels are low, you will feel weak. And if you don't have enough energy to really go after it during workouts, your fat-burning and muscle-building results will suffer, says Jim White, R.D., owner of Jim White Fitness and Nutrition Studios in Virginia.

How to Sweat Smart When Fasting

Does Fasted Cardio Burn More Fat?

Intermittent fasting enthusiasts don't need to throw in the towel on tough workouts just yet, though. Maintaining a consistent exercise routine is important for your health — both physical and mental. So if you're following an IF plan, here are the best ways to structure your workouts so you can still get great results:

1. Keep cardio low-intensity if you've been fasting.

A good gauge of intensity is your breathing: You should be able to carry on a conversation relatively easily if you're exercising mid-fast. "If you are going out for a light jog or stint on the elliptical, you probably aren't going to have an issue," says White. But it's important to listen to your body, and stop exercising, if you feel light-headed or dizzy. If you push your exercise intensity or duration too high, your workout will become a struggle.

2. Go high-intensity only after you've eaten.

Intermittent fasting programs like Lean Gains have strict rules about scheduling meals around workouts to maximize fat loss while still staying fueled. In general, the closer you schedule any moderate to intense sessions to your last meal, the better. That way you'll still have some glycogen (aka leftover carbs) available to fuel your workout, and you'll reduce your risk of low blood sugar levels, he says. Try to follow high-intensity workouts with a carb-rich snack, since your glycogen-tapped muscles will be hungry for more.

3. "Feast" on high-protein meals.

If you're looking to build serious muscle, you'll need to eat — both before and after lifting. While a pre-workout snack can help you fuel, regular protein consumption is vital to muscle synthesis both throughout the day and right after your strength workout, when your muscles are craving amino acids to repair themselves and grow, Pritchett says. To maximize muscle growth, the Academy of Nutrition and Dietetics recommends consuming 20 to 30 grams of high-quality protein every four hours while you are awake, including after training. On an IF plan, timing is key: Schedule your strength training workouts so that they're sandwiched between two meals, or at least two snacks. And make sure to use your "feast" meals to meet your protein needs.

4. Remember: Snacks are your friend.

Some IF plans allow dieters to eat both snacks and meals during their feast periods — so take advantage of that flexibility. A meal or snack consumed three to four hours before your workout (or one to two hours before, if you're prone to low blood sugar) will help ensure you have the energy to power through those reps. Aim for a meal that combines fast-acting carbohydrates with a blood sugar-stabilizing protein (like toast topped with peanut butter and banana slices). Within two hours of your last rep, chow down on a post-workout snack containing about 20 grams of protein and 20 grams of carbohydrates to promote muscle growth and help replete your glycogen stores so you stay energized, White says.

The fasted state produces two significant effects:

1. Improved insulin sensitivity. Put very simply, the body releases insulin (a hormone) when we eat to help us absorb the nutrients from our food. The hormone then takes the sugars out of our bloodstream and directs them to the liver, muscles, and fat cells to be used as energy later on. The trouble is that eating too much and too often can make us more resistant to insulin's effects, and while poor insulin sensitivity ups the risk of heart disease and cancer, it also makes it harder to lose body fat . Eating less freq uently (i.e. fasting more regularly) is one way to help remedy the issue, because it results in the body releasing insulin less often, so we become more sensitive to it—and that makes it easier to lose fat, improves blood flow to muscles, and even curbs the impact of an unhealthy diet .

2. The second reason a good old-fashioned fast can promote muscle gain and fat loss comes down to growth hormone (GH), a magical elixir of a hormone that helps the body make new muscle tissue, burn fat, and improve bone quality, physical function, and longevity . Along with regular weight training and proper sleep, fasting is one of the best ways to increase the body's GH: One study showed that 24 hours without food increases the male body's GH production by 2,000 freakin'percent, and 1,300 percent in women. The effect ends when the fast does, which is a compelling reason to fast regularly in order to keep muscle-friendly hormones at their highest levels.

We can't speak of muscle-friendly hormones without bringing up testosterone. Testosterone helps increase muscle mass and reduce body fat while also improving energy levels, boosting libido, and even combating depression and heart problems—in both men and women. Fasting alone may not have any effect on testosterone, but there is a surprisingly simple way to produce large amounts of both "T" and growth hormone at the same time, creating an optimal environment for building muscle and torching fat: Exercising while fasted.

The Fast Way to Improve Performance

Exercise, especially intense exercise that uses a lot of muscles (think compound movements like deadlifts and sq uats) causes a big surge in testosterone—which is why it can make good sense to combine exercise and fasting . Many studies have found that training in a fasted state is a terrific way to build lean mass and boost insulin sensitivity, not just because of the nifty hormonal responses, but also because it makes the body absorb the post-workout meal more efficiently.

Tuna and Egg Salad

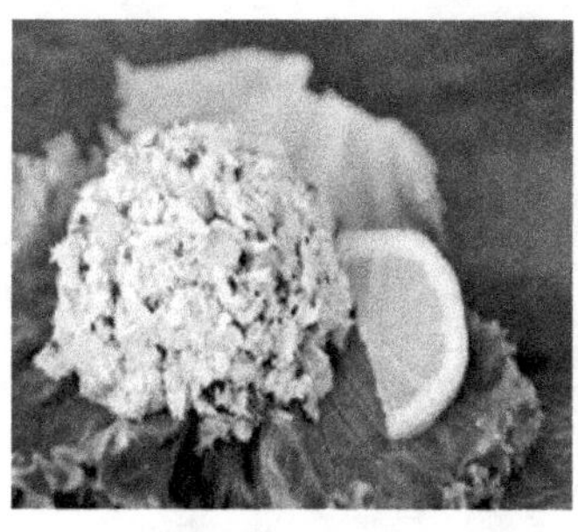

Ingredients:

4 egg whites, hard-boiled (68 calories)

1 egg, whole, hard-boiled (125 calories)

3 stalk celery, finely chopped (18 calories)

3 tbsp light mayo (105 calories)

¼ cup spring onions sliced finely or 3 stalks (14 calories)

1 x 185g / 6.5oz of canned tuna (in water, drained) (140 calories)

salt and freshly ground pepper for seasoning (0 calories)

a squeeze of lemon juice (1 calorie)

8 iceberg lettuce leaf cups (8 calories)

Preparation:

Take the hard boiled egg, egg whites, spring onions and celery in a chopper. Blitz or chop until finely diced.

Add seasoning, mayonnaise, lemon juice and a small pinch of paprika and combine all ingredients.

Let chill for about 2 hours so it's firm and holds shape.

Taking an iceberg lettuce peel off 8 leaves. Trim edges and use leaves as cups or wraps.

Take 2 lettuce leaves and ½ cup of tuna and egg mix and place in a lettuce cup, wrap and enjoy.

Calories: approx. 120 calories per serving

Servings: 4 (serving size 2 lettuce cups)

Sweet Potato and Chilli Soup

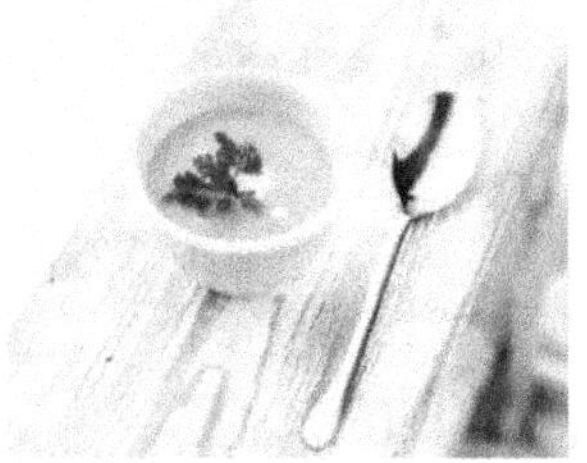

Ingredients:

1 tbsp vegetable oil (120 calories)

1 finely chopped medium onion (48 calories)

1 tbsp Chipotle / chilli paste (6 calories)

1 cube of vegetable stock (5 calories)

1.3L (5.5 cups) of boiling water (0 calories)

750g / 1.6lb sweet potatoes, peeled and cut into fine chunks or grated (645 calories)

Half/low-fat crème fraîche (15 calories)

Coriander/chives leaves

Method:

Heat the oil and fry off the onion until just soft, for about 4-5 mins, in a large saucepan. Add the paste and cook for 1 minute more.

In a separate container, add the boiling water and dissolve the stock cube. Then add to the pan, along with the sweet potato.

Bring back to the boil, then simmer for about 10 minutes, until the sweet potato is soft.

Puree the mixture with a stick blender until nice and smooth.

Ladle the soup mixture into serving bowls and add a dollop of crème fraîche, as well as a scattering of fresh coriander leaves and some chopped chives to garnish.

Calories: Total = 839 calories or 210 calories per serving

Servings: 4

Chicken and vegetable balti

Preparation time: less than 30 mins

Cooking time: 30 mins to 1 hour

Serves: Serves 2

Try this chicken and vegetable balti for a healthy curry that is q uick and easy to prepare.

As part of an Intermittent diet plan, 1 serving provides:

1 of your 3 daily low-fat dairy portions

2 of your 6 daily vegetable portions

This meal provides

341 kcal, 40g protein, 30.5g carbohydrate (of which 20.5g sugars), 6g fat (of which 1.5g saturates), 9g fibre and 0.6g salt per portion.

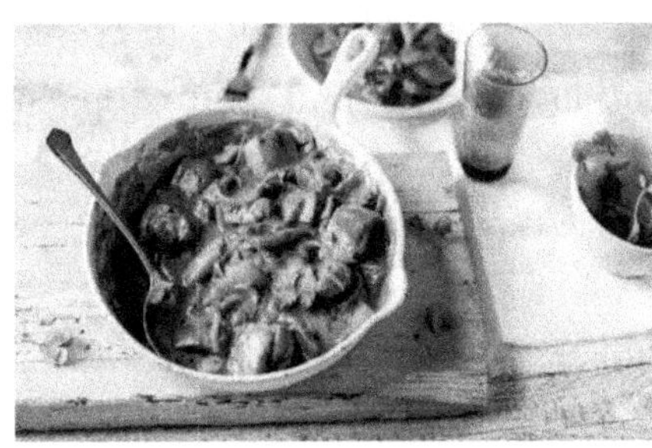

Ingredients

calorie controlled cooking oil spray

1 medium onion, thinly sliced

4 chicken thighs, boned and skinned

1 red pepper, deseeded and cut into 3cm/1in chunks

1 yellow pepper, deseeded and cut into 3cm/1in chunks

1 tbsp cornflour

150g/5½oz fat-free natural yogurt

1 tbsp medium or mild curry powder

2 garlic cloves, thinly sliced

227g/8oz tin chopped tomatoes

3 heaped tbsp finely chopped fresh coriander, plus extra to garnish

freshly ground black pepper

Method

Spray a large, deep, non-stick frying pan or wok with oil and place over a medium heat. Add the onion and cook for five minutes, stirring regularly until well softened and lightly browned.

Meanwhile, trim all the visible fat off the chicken thighs, cut each one into four pieces and season with black pepper.

Add the chicken and peppers into the pan with the onion and cook for three minutes, turning occasionally.

Meanwhile, in a small bowl, mix the cornflour with 2 tablespoons cold water and stir in the yoghurt until thoroughly mixed.

Sprinkle the curry powder over the chicken and vegetables, add the garlic and cook for 30 seconds.

Tip the tomatoes into the pan, add the yoghurt mixture, 150ml/3½fl oz of water and coriander.

Bring to a gentle simmer and cook for 20-25 minutes, stirring occasionally until the chicken is tender and the sauce is thick. Season with freshly ground black pepper to taste and garnish with coriander.

Garlic mushroom frittata

Preparation time:less than 30 mins

Cooking time: 10 to 30 mins

Serves: Serves 2

Garlic and mushrooms bring great flavour to this super-low-calorie, easy-to-make frittata. Serve with salad for a simple and delicious lunch.

As part of an Intermittent diet plan, 1 serving provides 3 of your 6 daily vegetable portions.

This meal provides

243 kcal, 14g protein, 3.5g carbohydrate (of which 3g sugars), 14g fat (of which 4g saturates), 2.5g fibre and 0.6g salt per portion.

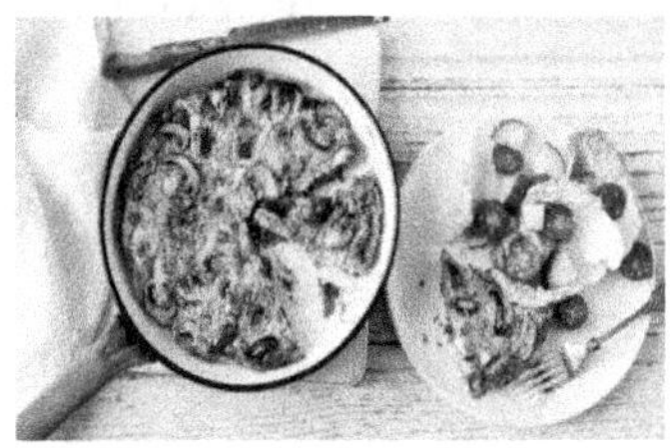

Ingredients

low-calorie cooking spray

250g/9oz chestnut mushrooms, sliced

1 small garlic clove, crushed

1 tbsp thinly sliced fresh chives

4 large free-range eggs, beaten

freshly ground black pepper

For the salad

1 Little Gem lettuce, leaves separated

100g/3½oz cherry tomatoes, halved

1/3 cucumber, cut into chunks

Method

Spray a small, flame-proof frying pan with oil and place over a high heat. (The base of the pan shouldn't be wider than about 18cm/7in.) Stir-fry the mushrooms in three batches for 2-3 minutes, or until softened and lightly browned. Tip the cooked mushrooms into a sieve over a bowl to catch any juices – you don't want the mushrooms to become soggy.

Return all the mushrooms to the pan and stir in the garlic and chives, and a pinch of ground black pepper. Cook for a further minute, then reduce the heat to low.

Preheat the grill to its hottest setting. Pour the eggs over the mushrooms. Cook for five minutes, or until almost set.

Place the pan under the grill for 3-4 minutes, or until set.

Combine the salad ingredients in a bowl.

Remove from the grill and loosen the sides of the frittata with a round-bladed knife. Turn out onto a board and cut into wedges. Serve hot or cold with the salad.

Extra-lean burger and salad

Preparation time: less than 30 mins

Cooking time: 10 to 30 mins

Serves: Serves 2

Forget fat-packed takeaway burgers. Tuck into our homemade 'fakeaway' treat.

As part of an Intermittent diet plan, 1 serving provides 2 of your 6 daily vegetable portions.

This meal provides

255 kcal, 36g protein, 6g carbohydrate (of which 5.5g sugars), 7g fat (of which 2.5g saturates), 3g fibre and 0.4g salt per portion.

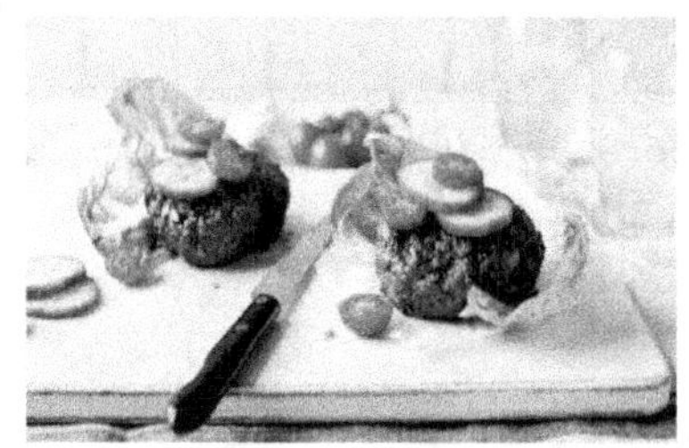

Ingredients

low-calorie cooking spray

½ small onion, finely chopped

100g/3½oz Portobello mushrooms, finely chopped

250g/9oz extra-lean beef mince (under 5% fat)

2 tsp finely chopped fresh thyme (or ½ tsp dried thyme)

freshly ground black pepper

For the salad

1 Little Gem lettuce, leaves separated

120g/4½oz cherry tomatoes, sliced

1/3 cucumber, sliced

Method

Spray a small frying pan with oil and cook the onion and mushrooms over a medium heat for five minutes, or until well softened, stirring regularly. Tip into a heatproof bowl and leave to cool for five minutes.

Add the beef, thyme and lots of ground black pepper. Mix well and form into two balls. Flatten into burger shapes, each around 2cm/¾in thick.

Clean the pan and return to the hob. Spray with a little more oil and cook the burgers over a medium-low heat for 10 minutes, turning occasionally, until browned on the outside and cooked through inside.

Serve the burgers with lettuce, tomatoes and cucumber.

Lamb and flageolet bean stew

Preparation time: less than 30 mins

Cooking time: 1 to 2 hours

Serves: Serves 4

This is a warming stew perfect for filling you up on a cold evening. Don't be put off by the long cooking time, this is an easy one-pot supper that will reward you for your patience.

As part of an Intermittent diet plan, 1 serving provides:

- your daily salty food

- 3 of your 6 daily vegetable portions

This meal provides 288 kcal per portion.

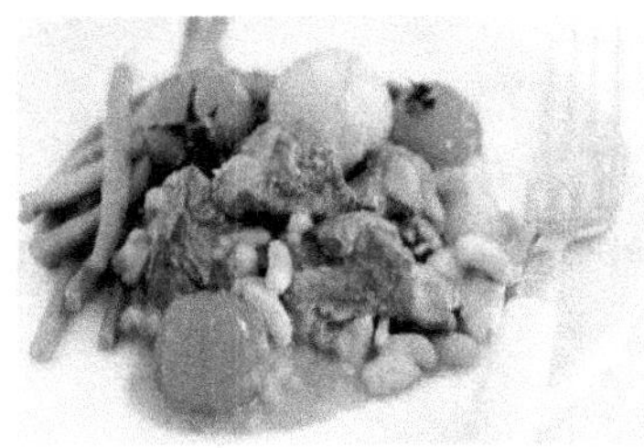

Ingredients

1 tsp olive oil

350g/12oz lean lamb, cubed

16 pickling onions

1 garlic clove, crushed

600ml/20fl oz lamb stock (made with concentrated liq uid stock)

200g can chopped tomatoes

1 bouq uet garni

2 x 400g cans flageolet beans, drained and rinsed

320g/11oz green beans

250g/9oz cherry tomatoes

freshly ground black pepper

Method

Heat the oil in a flameproof casserole or saucepan, add the lamb and fry for 3-4 minutes until browned all over. Remove the lamb from the casserole and set aside.

Add the onions and garlic to the pan and fry for 4-5 minutes, or until the onions are beginning to brown.

Return the lamb and any juices to the pan. Add the stock, tomatoes, bouq uet garni and beans. Bring to the boil, stirring, then cover and simmer for 1 hour, or until the lamb is just tender.

Meanwhile, bring a pan of water to the boil and blanch the green beans. Place in bowl of ice-cold water.

Add the cherry tomatoes to the stew and season well with freshly ground black pepper. Continue to simmer for 10 minutes.

Divide the stew between four plates, place the green beans alongside and serve.

Cinnamon porridge with grated pear

Preparation time: less than 30 mins

Cooking time: less than 10 mins

Serves: Serves 2

This porridge is made with water and skimmed milk to keep the calories low. A little ground cinnamon makes it taste sweeter without adding calories and it is topped with juicy grated pear.

As part of an Intermittent diet plan, 1 serving provides a half portion of your 6 daily vegetable portions, 1 of your dairy portions and 219 kcal.

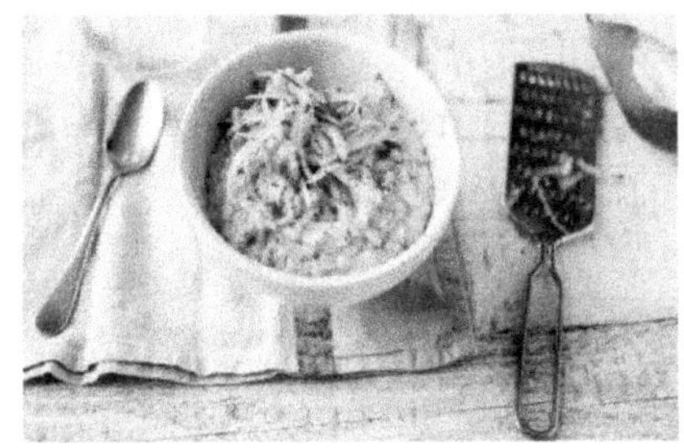

Ingredients

60g/2¼oz jumbo porridge oats

¼ tsp ground cinnamon, plus a little to sprinkle

300ml/10fl oz semi-skimmed milk

1 ripe medium pear

1 wedge lemon

Method

Put the oats and cinnamon in a non-stick saucepan with the milk and cook over a low-medium heat for 4-5 minutes, stirring constantly until rich and creamy. Pour into two deep bowls.

Coarsely grate the pear, and place on top of the porridge. Sq ueeze over the lemon juice and sprinkle with a tiny pinch of ground cinnamon.

Peppered beef with salad leaves

Preparation time: less than 30 mins

Cooking time: less than 10 mins

Serves: Serves 2

This is a speedy supper, perfect for a busy evening. Horseradish sauce adds a kick to the salad dressing.

As part of an Intermittent diet plan, 1 serving provides 1 of your 6 daily vegetable portions and 148 kcal.

If eating it as part of a daily Intermittent diet menu, also enjoy a piece of fruit with this meal (about 70 calories).

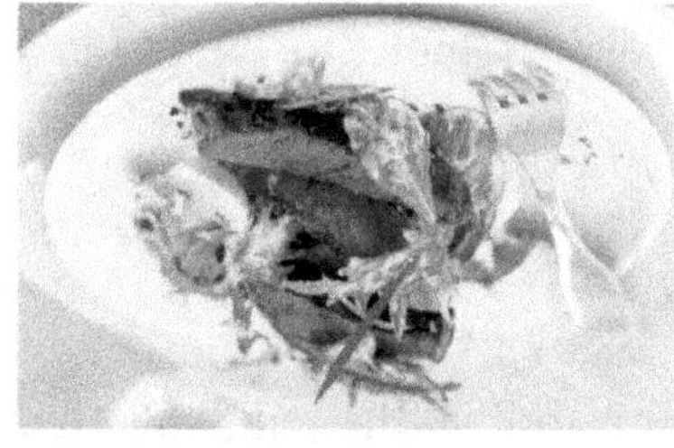

Ingredients

2 thick-cut sirloin steaks, about 175g/6oz in total, fat trimmed

1 tsp coloured peppercorns, coarsely crushed

coarse salt flakes

60g/2¼oz natural yoghurt

½ tsp horseradish sauce (to taste)

½ garlic clove, crushed

50g/2oz mixed green salad leaves

30g/1¼oz button mushrooms, sliced

½ red onion, thinly sliced

1 tsp olive oil

salt and freshly ground black pepper

Method

Rub the steaks with the crushed peppercorns and salt flakes.

Mix together the yoghurt, horseradish sauce and garlic and season to taste with salt and freshly ground black pepper. Add the salad leaves, mushrooms and most of the red onion and toss gently.

Heat the oil in a frying pan, add the steaks and cook over a high heat for 2 minutes, or until browned. Turn over and cook for a further 2 minutes for medium rare, 3-4 minutes for medium or 5 minutes for well done. Place the steak on a warm plate and allow to rest for a few minutes.

Spoon the salad leaves into the centre of 2 serving plates. Thinly slice the steaks and arrange the pieces on top. Garnish with the remaining red onion.

Caponata ratatouille

Preparation time: less than 30 mins

Cooking time: 30 mins to 1 hour

Serves: Serves 6

Ratatouille is a wonderfully warming vegetable stew originating from Provence. Perfect for pleasing vegetarians and meat-eaters alike.

As part of an Intermittent diet plan, 1 serving provides:

Your daily salty food

2 of your 6 daily vegetable portions

This meal provides 90 kcal per portion.

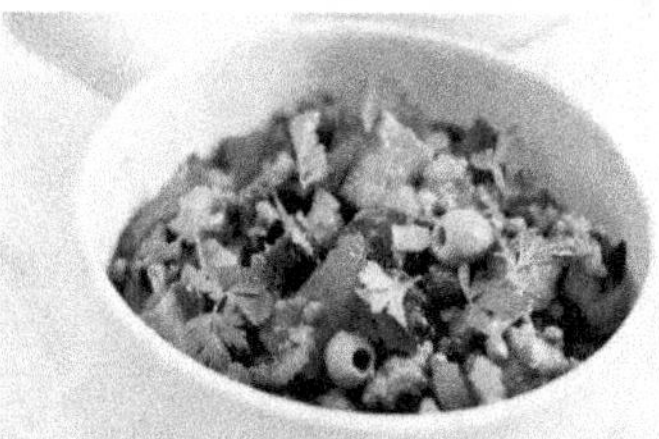

Ingredients

1 tbsp olive oil

750g/1lb 10oz aubergines, cut into 1cm/1½in chunks

1 large onion, cut into 1cm/1½in chunks

3 celery sticks, roughly chopped

2 large beef tomatoes, skinned and deseeded

1 tsp chopped thyme

¼-½ tsp cayenne pepper

2 tbsp capers, drained

small handful pitted green olives

4 tbsp white wine vinegar

1 tbsp sugar

1-2 tbsp cocoa powder (optional)

freshly ground black pepper

To garnish

chopped almonds, toasted

chopped parsley

Recipe tips

Method

Heat the oil in a non-stick frying pan until very hot, add the aubergine and fry for about 15 minutes, or until very soft. Add a little boiling water to prevent sticking if necessary.

Meanwhile, place the onion and celery in a large saucepan with a little water. Cook for 5 minutes, or until tender but still firm.

Add the tomatoes, thyme, cayenne pepper and aubergine to the saucepan. Cook for 15 minutes, stirring occasionally. Add the capers, olives, vinegar, sugar and cocoa powder and cook for 2-3 minutes.

Season with freshly ground black pepper. Divide between 6 bowls, garnish with the toasted almonds and parsley and serve.

Moroccan baked eggs

Preparation time: less than 30 mins

Cooking time: 10 to 30 mins

Serves: Serves 2

Baked eggs are the perfect dish for a lazy brunch. If you like your eggs spicy just add a little chilli powder.

As part of an Intermittent diet plan, 1 serving provides 2 of your 6 daily vegetable portions.

This meal provides 170 kcal per portion. If eating it as part of a daily Intermittent diet menu, also enjoy 200ml skimmed milk (70 calories).

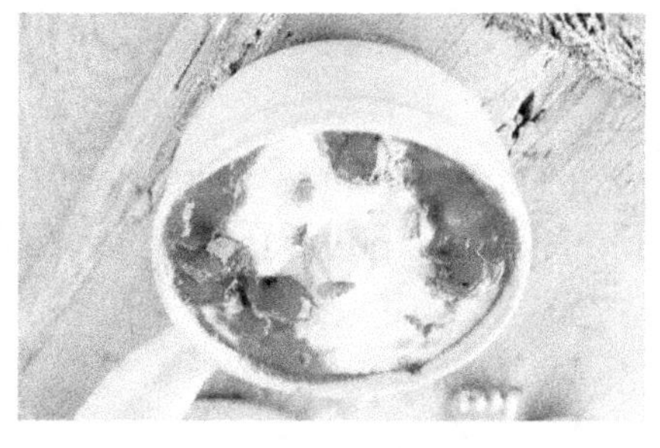

Ingredients

  ½ tbsp olive oil

  ½ onion, chopped

  1 garlic clove, sliced

  ½ tsp ras-el-hanout

pinch ground cinnamon

½ tsp ground coriander

400g/14oz cherry tomatoes, chopped

2 tbsp chopped coriander

2 free-range eggs

salt and freshly ground black pepper

Method

Preheat the oven to 220C/200C Fan/Gas 7.

Heat the oil in a frying pan, add the onion and garlic and cook for 6-7 minutes, or until soft. Stir in the spices and cook, stirring, for a further minute.

Add the tomatoes and season well with salt and pepper, then simmer gently for 8-10 minutes.

Scatter over 1 tablespoon of the coriander, then divide the tomato mixture between 2 individual ovenproof dishes. Break an egg into each dish.

Bake for 8-10 minutes until the egg whites are set but the yolks are still slightly runny. Cook for a further 2-3 minutes if you prefer the eggs to be cooked through.

Scatter over the remaining coriander and serve.

Vegetables with red pepper rouille

Preparation time: 30 mins to 1 hour

Cooking time: 30 mins to 1 hour

Serves: Serves 6

Roasted vegetables do not have to be boring, flavour with saffron and serve with a smoky red pepper rouille to create a tasty vegetarian supper.

For this recipe you will need a liq uidizer or food processor.

As part of an Intermittent diet plan, 1 serving provides 2 of your 6 daily vegetable portions.

This meal provides 142 kcal per portion.

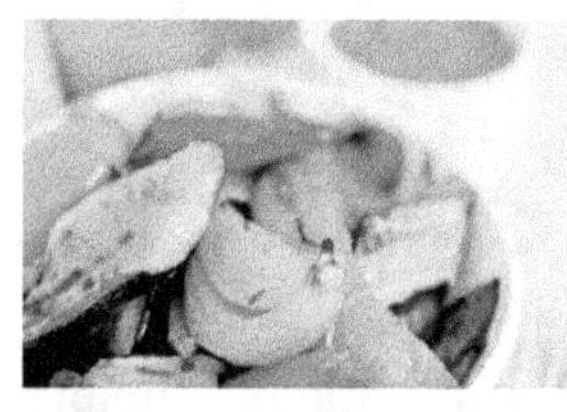

Ingredients

4 tbsp olive oil

2-3 garlic cloves, finely chopped

3 large pinches of saffron threads

3 mixed red and orange peppers, cored, deseeded and each cut into 6 strips

3 courgettes, about 100g/3½oz each, chopped into 2.5cm/1in chunks

2 onions, cut into wedges

salt and freshly ground black pepper

For the rouille

4 plum tomatoes, about 250g/9oz in total

1 red pepper, cored, deseeded and quartered

1 garlic clove, finely chopped

large pinch of ground smoked paprika

1 tbsp olive oil

Method

Preheat the oven to 220C/200C Fan/Gas 7.

Put the oil for the vegetables in a large plastic bag with the garlic, saffron and some salt and pepper. Add the vegetables, grip the top edge of the bag to seal and toss together. Set aside for at least 30 minutes.

Meanwhile for the rouille, put the tomatoes and pepper in a small roasting tin. Sprinkle with the garlic, smoked paprika some salt and pepper. Then drizzle the oil over and roast for 15 minutes. Allow to cool.

Peel the skins from the tomatoes and pepper. Purée the flesh in a liquidizer or food processor with any juices from the roasting tin until smooth. Spoon into a serving bowl and set aside, keep warm.

Tip the saffron vegetables into a large roasting tin and cook in the oven for 15-20 minutes, turning once, until browned.

Spoon the vegetables on to individual plates and serve with spoonfuls of the rouille.

Chilli and coriander fish parcel

Preparation time: 1-2 hours

Cooking time: 10 to 30 mins

Serves: Serves 1

Baking fish is a great way to reduce calories. Give the fish extra oomph with chilli and coriander.

For this recipe you will need a blender or a food processor.

As part of an Intermittent diet plan, 1 serving provides 1 of your 6 daily vegetable portions and 148 calories.

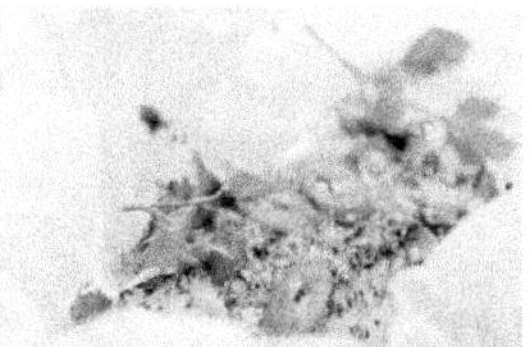

Ingredients

125g/4½oz cod, coley or haddock fillet

2 tsp lemon juice

1 tbsp fresh coriander leaves

1 garlic clove, roughly chopped

1 green chilli, deseeded and chopped

¼ tsp sugar

2 tsp natural yoghurt

80g/3oz mangetout, steamed, to serve

Method

Preheat the oven to 200C/180C Fan/Gas 6.

Place the fish in a non-metallic dish and sprinkle with the lemon juice. Cover and leave in the fridge to marinate for 15-20 minutes.

Put the coriander, garlic and chilli in a food processor or blender and process until the mixture forms a paste. Add the sugar and yoghurt and briefly process to blend.

Lay the fish on a sheet of foil. Coat the fish on both sides with the paste. Gather up the foil loosely and turn over at the top to seal. Return to the fridge for at least 1 hour.

Place the parcel on a baking tray and bake for about 15 minutes, or until the fish is just cooked. Serve with the mangetout.

Warm chicken salad

Preparation time: less than 30 mins

Cooking time: 10 to 30 mins

Serves: Serves 2

A gorgeous chicken salad that can be served warm or cold, perfect for a quick healthy supper.

As part of an Intermittent diet plan, 1 serving provides 2 of your 6 daily vegetable portions.

This meal provides 205 kcal per portion.

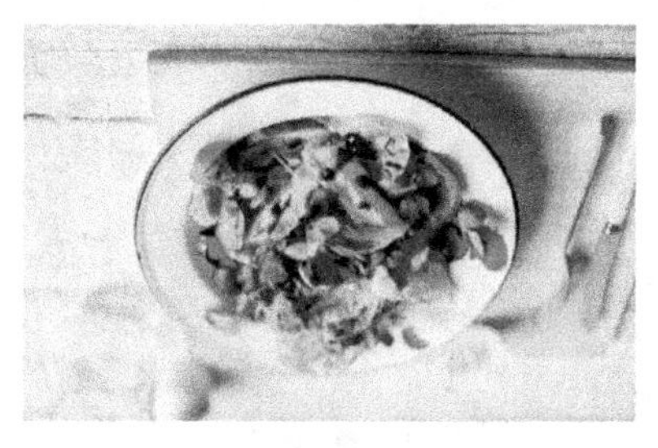

Ingredients

2 small chicken breasts, boned, skinned and cut in half

calorie controlled cooking oil spray

1 large orange or red pepper, deseeded and cut in to chunks

1 little gem lettuce, leaves separated

50g/1¾oz watercress, tough stalks removed

2 ripe medium tomatoes, cut into small chunks

? cucumber, sliced

1 tsp thick balsamic vinegar

½ small lemon, juice only

sea salt and freshly ground black pepper

Method

Season the chicken pieces on both sides with salt and pepper. Spray a large non-stick frying pan with oil and place over a high heat. Cook the chicken pieces for three minutes on each side or until lightly browned and cooked through. Transfer to a plate.

Spray the pan with a little more oil and cook the pepper for three minutes on each side or until lightly charred and beginning to soften.

Arrange the lettuce leaves, watercress, tomatoes, cucumber and pepper on two plates.

Slice the chicken breasts and scatter on top of salad. Drizzle with the balsamic vinegar and squeeze the lemon juice over. Season with black pepper and serve.

Thank you!